TABLE OF CONTENTS

Chapter 1

Introduction

Rediscovering the Healing Wisdom of Nature with Jigsimur

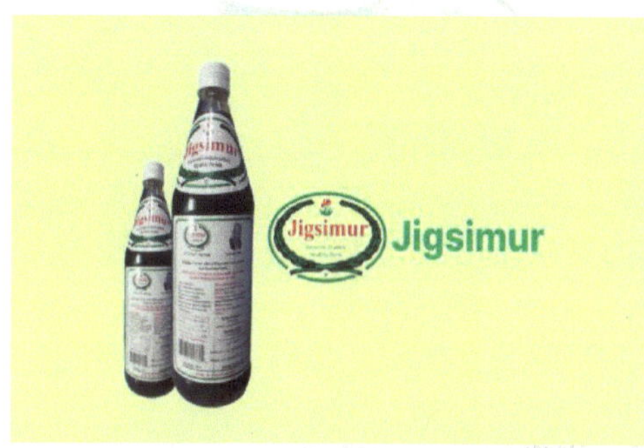

In an age defined by rapid technological improvements and the consistent pursuit of progress, there's a quiet and profound yearning to return to the embrace of nature. The alluring charm of natural remedies, drawn from the Earth's bounty, has captured the imagination of many seeking a holistic approach to health and wellness. Amid this resurgence of interest, one remarkable herbal solution shines brightly—Jigsimur.

Nature's wisdom has been cultivated for millennia by indigenous cultures across the globe, and Jigsimur stands as a testament to the potency of these ancient traditions. In the pages of this ebook, "Jigsimur: Nature's Treasure for Health and Wellness," we embark on a journey to unravel the mysteries surrounding this remarkable gift from the natural world.

A Legacy Rooted in Tradition

Jigsimur, with its roots deeply entwined in the history of traditional African medicine, encapsulates generations of wisdom passed down through time. The art of healing through plants, revered by ancestral healers, forms the foundation of Jigsimur's origins. This herbal remedy, a testament to cultural heritage, draws its name from the combination of "jig" (meaning "harmful things" in Hausa) and "simur" (meaning "throw away" in Yoruba)—a symbolic representation of its power to discard what is harmful and restore balance.

Exploring Nature's Pharmacy

The composition of Jigsimur is a symphony of nature's finest offerings. An ensemble of carefully selected botanical ingredients combines to create a holistic powerhouse that offers a range of health benefits. As we delve deeper into this ebook, we will embark on a journey to unveil the unique properties and potential effects of each component, gaining insights into their synergistic interactions that add to Jigsimur's remarkable efficacy.

Beyond Symptoms: A Holistic Approach

At the core of Jigsimur's philosophy is the recognition that health is not merely the absence of illness but a harmonious balance between mind, body, and spirit. As we explore the numerous health benefits of Jigsimur, we'll also discover its role in addressing chronic conditions and advancing overall well-being. With its potential to enhance digestion, support the immune system, detoxify the body, and nourish joints and bones, Jigsimur presents a comprehensive approach to health that resonates deeply with those seeking natural solutions.

Bridging Tradition and Science

While rooted in ancient traditions, Jigsimur's story doesn't stop at the pages of history. Modern science has begun to unravel the mechanisms behind its efficacy, bridging the gap between traditional wisdom and contemporary understanding. Throughout this ebook, we'll explore the ongoing research and scientific insights that shed light on Jigsimur's cellular interactions and therapeutic potential.

Embarking on a Personal Journey

As you read through the chapters that follow, you'll encounter testimonials of individuals whose lives have been touched by the healing grace of Jigsimur. Their stories offer glimpses into the profound transformations that can arise when nature's treasures are harnessed with intention and respect.

In the pages ahead, we invite you to embrace the wisdom of generations past, align with the healing forces of nature, and embark on a journey of discovery that might just redefine your understanding of health and wellness. Welcome to "Jigsimur: Nature's Treasure for Health and Wellness."

Chapter 2

The Origins of Jigsimur

Historical Echoes: Unearthing the Roots of Jigsimur

In the heart of the African continent, where traditions are woven into the fabric of daily life, a remarkable herbal remedy called Jigsimur has flourished for centuries. The history of Jigsimur is a tapestry of wisdom, culture, and healing, woven by generations past and held sacred by those who recognize its extraordinary potential.

The tale of Jigsimur finds its beginnings in the traditions of indigenous African healers, who crafted their knowledge of the natural world into remedies that addressed ailments of both body and spirit. Passed down through generations, this legacy of healing eventually culminated in the creation of Jigsimur—an embodiment of ancient wisdom made accessible to the modern world.

Tradition's Embrace: Jigsimur's Role in African Culture

The significance of Jigsimur extends far beyond its medicinal properties; it is an integral part of African culture, symbolizing the reverence for nature and the interconnectedness of all living things. In various African societies, the role of healers and medicine men was pivotal, and their ability to harness the healing properties of plants was considered a divine gift.

Jigsimur, named as a testament to its power to expel harmful elements and restore equilibrium, was a central fixture in the practices of these revered healers. Its incorporation into rituals, ceremonies, and daily life marked it not only as a remedy but also as a bridge between the physical and spiritual realms. This cultural resonance elevated Jigsimur to a position of honor, where its efficacy was celebrated in the same breath as the traditions it sprung from.

Nature's Bounty: The Ingredients That Shape Jigsimur

At the heart of Jigsimur's efficacy lies a carefully curated selection of botanical treasures, each chosen for its unique properties and synergistic

potential. This combination of natural ingredients serves as a testament to the nuanced understanding of the intricate balance within the body and the environment.

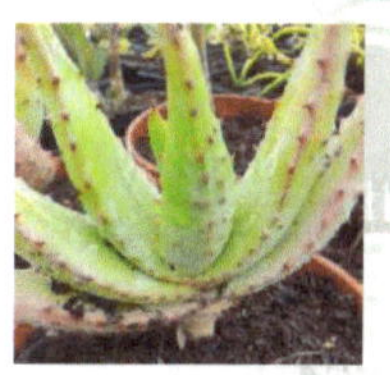

1. Aloe Ferox: A cornerstone of Jigsimur, Aloe Ferox boasts an array of bioactive compounds that suppliment to its healing properties. Renowned for its anti-inflammatory and detoxifying effects, Aloe Ferox supports digestive health and helps rid the body of toxins that can impede wellness.

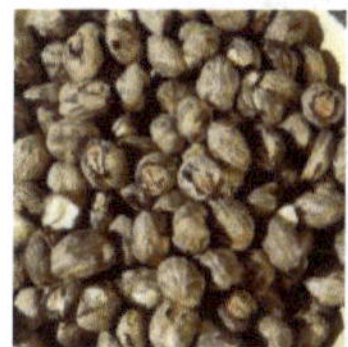

2. Mongongo Nut: Extracted from the Mongongo tree, this nut is rich in essential fatty acids, antioxidants, and vitamins. It add s to Jigsimur's ability to nourish joints, bones, and skin, nurturing overall vitality.

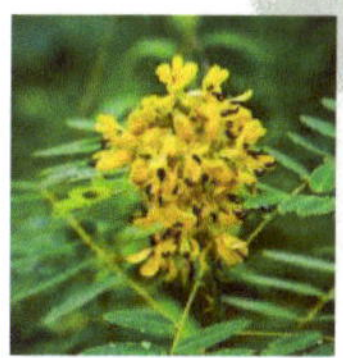

3. Senna Plant: Recognized for its gentle laxative effects, the Senna plant adds a digestive component to Jigsimur's comprehensive benefits. It supports natural bowel movement and aids in detoxification.

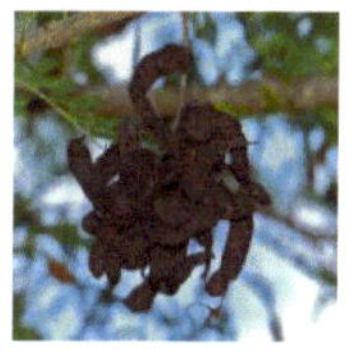

4. Sickle Bush: The Sickle Bush's potent anti-inflammatory properties enhance Jigsimur's potential to soothe joint discomfort and promote overall immune health.

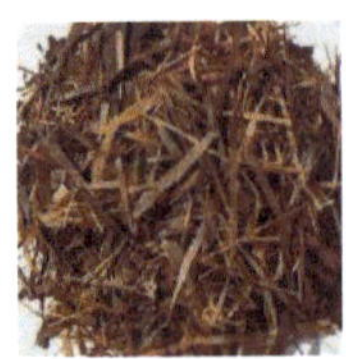

5. Pau D'arco: With its antimicrobial and immune-boosting qualities, Pau D'arco complements Jigsimur's holistic approach by fostering a robust defense against external threats.

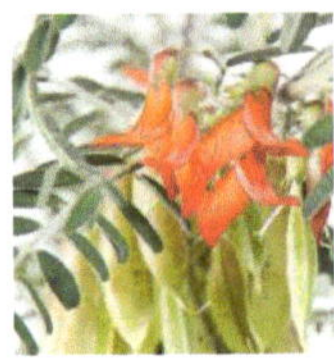

6. Sutherlandia Frutescens: Known for its adaptogenic properties, Sutherlandia Frutescens supports the body's stress response and helps maintain balance during periods of challenge.

Cultivating Curiosity: A Journey Begins

The origins of Jigsimur are a testament to the wisdom and insight of those who understood the harmonious relationship between nature and well-being. In the chapters ahead, we'll explore not only the historical roots and cultural significance of Jigsimur but also the intricate science that underpins its remarkable effects. As we embark on this journey, let us remember that every drop of Jigsimur carries with it the legacy of generations past, a testament to the enduring quest for health, harmony, and connection.

Chapter 3

Unveiling the Composition

Analyzing the Components of Jigsimur: Nature's Symphony of Healing

As we delve deeper into the heart of Jigsimur, we embark on an exploration of its intricate composition—an assembly of nature's finest components synergistically woven together to create a powerhouse of health and wellness. Each ingredient is a note in a symphony, contributing its unique melody to the harmony that is Jigsimur.

1. Aloe Ferox: The Healing Elixir

Aloe Ferox takes center stage in Jigsimur's composition. Its gel-like substance is a reservoir of vitamins, minerals, enzymes, and amino acids that collectively donate to its healing potential. This ingredient's anti-inflammatory and antioxidant properties are key players in soothing digestive discomfort and improving overall well-being.

2. Mongongo Nut: The Nutrient-Rich Gem

The Mongongo nut offers a bounty of essential nutrients, including linoleic acid and vitamin E. These components nourish the body from within, enhancing skin health, joint mobility, and cardiovascular wellness. Its presence in Jigsimur donate s to its multi-faceted approach to holistic health.

3. Senna Plant: Gentle Detoxification

The Senna plant's leaves contain compounds known as anthraquinones, which gently stimulate the bowels and promote healthy digestion. This aspect of Jigsimur aids in the body's natural detoxification process, ensuring that waste and toxins are efficiently eliminated.

4. Sickle Bush: Soothing Inflammation

The Sickle Bush, rich in flavonoids and phenolic compounds, is a natural anti-inflammatory agent. Its presence in Jigsimur add s to the remedy's potential to alleviate joint discomfort and support a healthy immune response.

5. Pau D'arco: Defense and Vitality

Pau D'arco's lapachol content provides it with antimicrobial and immune-boosting properties. This ingredient strengthens Jigsimur's ability to shield the body from external threats while improving overall vitality.

6. Sutherlandia Frutescens: Adaptogenic Elegance

Sutherlandia Frutescens, known as an adaptogen, helps the body manage stress and maintain balance. Its inclusion in Jigsimur ensures that the remedy addresses both physical and emotional aspects of well-being.

Phytochemicals and Their Potential Effects: Nature's Arsenal of Wellness

Phytochemicals, the naturally occurring compounds in plants, are the biochemical artisans responsible for Jigsimur's remarkable effects. Flavonoids, terpenoids, polyphenols, and alkaloids are just a few examples of these potent molecules that donate to Jigsimur's therapeutic prowess. These compounds interact with the body on a cellular level, influencing processes that range from inflammation regulation to cellular repair.

Synergy Among Ingredients for Enhanced Benefits: The Whole is Greater Than the Sum

What sets Jigsimur apart is not just the individual contributions of its ingredients, but the synergy that emerges when these components unite. The combined effects of Aloe Ferox's anti-inflammatory properties, the Mongongo nut's nourishing capabilities, and the Senna plant's gentle detoxification create a holistic approach to wellness that surpasses what each ingredient could achieve alone. This harmony is a testament to the wisdom of nature, where the collective strength of the parts elevates the whole.

As we peel back the layers of Jigsimur's composition, we witness the symphony of healing taking shape. The intricate dance of phytochemicals and the collaborative spirit of nature's bounty lay the groundwork for the transformative effects that await us. In the upcoming chapters, we'll delve into the health benefits that emerge from this symphony, understanding how each note donate s to the melody of well-being.

Chapter 4

Health Benefits of Jigsimur

Nature's Elixir: Unlocking the Multifaceted Health Benefits of Jigsimur

As we continue our exploration of Jigsimur's remarkable potential, we venture into the realm of its health benefits—a comprehensive array of wellness advantages that cater to the body's intricate systems. Jigsimur's synergy of natural ingredients is a testament to the profound healing capacities of nature.

1. Digestive System Support: A Harmonious Balance

The digestive system is the gateway to overall health, and Jigsimur stands as a guardian of its equilibrium. The Aloe Ferox in Jigsimur holds a special place in this role. With its anti-inflammatory properties and soothing effects, it can help alleviate gastrointestinal discomfort, support healthy bowel movement, and promote a balanced digestive environment.

2. Immune System Enhancement: Fortifying Defenses

The immune system is the body's sentinel, defending against external threats. Jigsimur's multifaceted composition, enriched with immune-enhancing elements like Pau D'arco and Sickle Bush, fortifies the body's defenses against infections, improving resilience and overall well-being.

3. Detoxification and Cleansing Properties: Nature's Purification Ritual

Detoxification is an essential aspect of maintaining health in the modern world. Jigsimur, through the inclusion of Senna plant and Aloe Ferox, aids the body's natural detoxification processes. These ingredients gently encourage the elimination of waste, ensuring that toxins are expelled, and the body can function optimally.

4. Joint and Bone Health Promotion: Nourishing Vital Mobility

Jigsimur's influence extends to the musculoskeletal system, where it offers support for joints and bones. The Mongongo nut, with its wealth of essential fatty acids, add s to the nourishment of joints, improving flexibility and comfort. As we age, the maintenance of joint health becomes crucial, and Jigsimur's holistic approach offers a natural solution.

5. Cardiovascular System Benefits: Nurturing Heart Health

The cardiovascular system is the engine that powers life itself, and Jigsimur's ingredients work harmoniously to nurture its health. With its anti-inflammatory and antioxidant components, Jigsimur add s to a healthy heart by supporting blood vessel function and circulation. The combined effects of the remedy's ingredients can help maintain healthy blood pressure and cholesterol levels.

Holistic Wellness: A Tapestry of Benefits

The beauty of Jigsimur's health benefits lies in their interconnectedness—a symphony of effects that resonate across multiple systems of the body. As the digestive, immune, detoxification, joint, and cardiovascular systems experience improvements, they create a harmonious cascade that enhances overall well-being.

In the upcoming chapters, we'll dive even deeper into the specific conditions where Jigsimur shines, exploring its potential in managing chronic conditions and alleviating discomfort. From diabetes management to arthritis relief, Jigsimur's multifaceted benefits prove that nature's treasure chest is filled with answers for those seeking a holistic path to health and wellness.

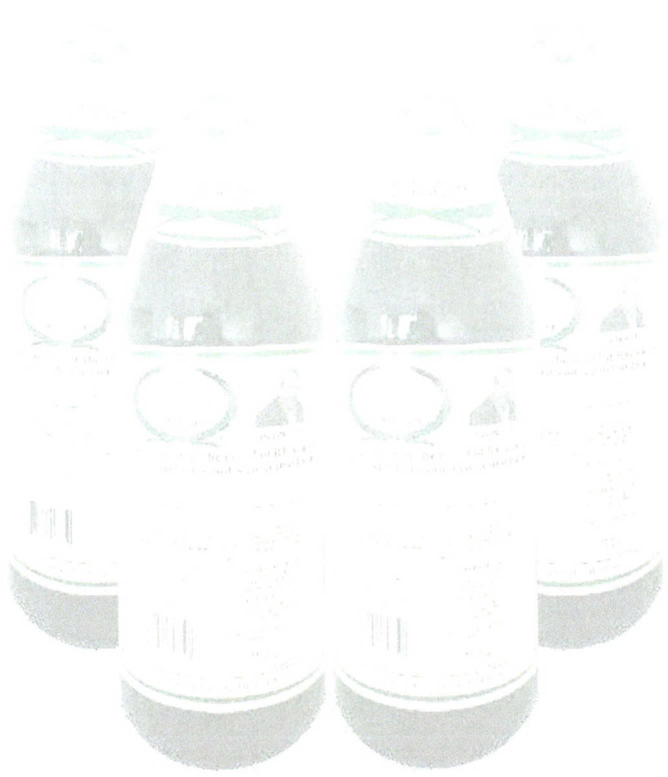

Chapter 5

Jigsimur and Chronic Conditions

Empowering Wellness: Jigsimur's Impact on Chronic Conditions

As we journey deeper into the world of Jigsimur, we uncover its potential to address chronic conditions—a testament to its holistic approach to health and wellness. Beyond its general benefits, Jigsimur's unique composition lends itself to aiding those managing specific health challenges, providing a ray of hope and relief.

1. Role in Managing Diabetes: A Natural Ally

Diabetes is a chronic condition that requires careful management of blood sugar levels. Jigsimur steps in as a natural ally in this journey. With its blend of ingredients, including Aloe Ferox and Pau D'arco, Jigsimur may play a role in stabilizing blood sugar levels, enhancing insulin sensitivity, and supporting overall metabolic health.

2. Impact on Blood Pressure and Cholesterol: Nurturing Cardiovascular Wellness

A healthy cardiovascular system is essential for overall well-being, and Jigsimur's influence extends to maintaining heart health. The remedy's components, such as Sickle Bush and Aloe Ferox, are known for their potential to regulate blood pressure and cholesterol levels. By fostering the integrity of blood vessels and supporting proper circulation, Jigsimur supplies to cardiovascular vitality.

3. Arthritis Relief and Joint Mobility Improvement: Easing the Path to Movement

Arthritis, with its often-debilitating effects on joint health, is a condition that significantly impacts quality of life. Jigsimur's multifaceted composition, including the joint-nourishing Mongongo nut and the anti-inflammatory

Sickle Bush, offers a ray of hope for individuals seeking relief from joint discomfort. By addressing inflammation and improving joint mobility, Jigsimur plays a role in enhancing the quality of life for those dealing with arthritis.

A Path to Empowerment: Holistic Wellness for Chronic Conditions

The chronic conditions discussed in this chapter share a common thread—they require a comprehensive approach to management. Jigsimur's holistic philosophy aligns perfectly with this need, offering a blend of ingredients that work in harmony to address various aspects of health. By empowering individuals with natural tools for managing chronic conditions, Jigsimur stands as a beacon of hope for those seeking a more holistic path to wellness.

In the upcoming chapters, we'll dive even further into the scientific insights behind Jigsimur's effects, exploring the mechanisms that underlie its impact on these chronic conditions. As we unravel the complexities of Jigsimur's interactions with the body, we'll gain a deeper appreciation for its potential to transform lives and promote enduring well-being.

Chapter 6

Incorporating Jigsimur into Your Routine

Embracing Nature's Bounty: A Practical Guide to Integrate Jigsimur into Your Lifestyle

As you embark on your journey to wellness with Jigsimur, this chapter serves as your compass, guiding you through the essential steps of seamlessly incorporating this natural treasure into your daily routine. With careful consideration, balance, and mindfulness, you can make Jigsimur an integral part of your holistic health journey.

1. Proper Dosage and Usage Guidelines: A Blueprint for Success

Understanding the appropriate dosage and usage of Jigsimur is the cornerstone of its effectiveness. Every individual is unique, and factors such as age, health condition, and wellness goals play a role in determining the ideal dosage. Start by referring to the product's packaging for recommended dosages. It's important to initiate your journey with the suggested amount and allow your body time to acclimate.

2. Precautions and Potential Side Effects: Navigating with Awareness

While Jigsimur is a natural solution, it's crucial to approach its integration into your routine with mindfulness. Before introducing it, consult with a healthcare professional, especially if you have existing health conditions or are taking medications. Although side effects are rare, some individuals may experience mild digestive discomfort initially. Monitoring your body's response and adjusting the dosage if necessary ensures a positive experience.

3. Combining Jigsimur with a Balanced Lifestyle: Synergy for Optimal Wellness

Jigsimur's potential is magnified when it collaborates with a balanced lifestyle. While its benefits are significant, it's essential to view it as a component of a holistic approach. Encompassing regular physical activity, a nourishing diet, adequate hydration, effective stress management, and ample sleep, a balanced lifestyle provides the foundation upon which Jigsimur's effects can flourish.

Seamless Integration: Steps to Weave Jigsimur into Your Routine

1. Start with Intent: Set clear intentions for your wellness journey with Jigsimur. Define your health goals and how you envision its role in achieving them.

2. Timing is Key: Determine the optimal time to incorporate Jigsimur into your daily routine. Whether it's before meals or at a specific time of day, consistency is key.

3. Begin Gradually: Commence with the recommended dosage, allowing your body to adapt. Gradually adjust the dosage as you monitor your body's response.

4. Hydration Support: Adequate hydration amplifies the effects of Jigsimur. Make water an integral part of your routine.

5. Lifestyle Synergy: Combine Jigsimur with a well-rounded lifestyle that embraces movement, nutrition, rest, stress management, and social connection.

6. Listen to Your Body: Your body communicates its needs and reactions. Pay attention to how you feel, and make adjustments as necessary.

A Harmonious Journey: Blending Jigsimur with Your Life

Incorporating Jigsimur into your daily routine is a commitment to nurturing your well-being. By fusing nature's wisdom with your personal wellness goals and embracing a balanced lifestyle, you embark on a harmonious journey of transformation. As we proceed with our exploration, let the integration of Jigsimur into your life serve as a testament to the profound alignment between nature's treasures and your quest for holistic health..

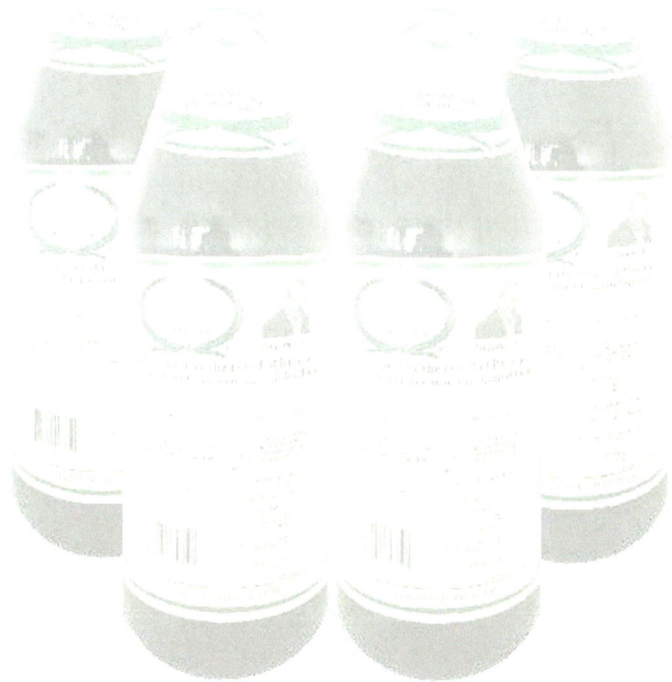

Chapter 7

Research and Scientific Insights

Unveiling the Science: Exploring Jigsimur's Impact through Research and Understanding

This chapter invites you to delve into the world of research and scientific exploration that sheds light on the inner workings of Jigsimur. As we uncover the evidence behind its effects, we bridge the gap between ancient wisdom and modern knowledge, painting a comprehensive picture of its potential for health and wellness.

1. Studies on Jigsimur's Effectiveness: A Glimpse into Research

The journey to understanding Jigsimur's impact begins with scientific studies that validate its effectiveness. Over time, numerous research endeavors have sought to unveil the mysteries of this natural treasure. Clinical trials, laboratory experiments, and observational studies provide insights into how Jigsimur influences health and wellness. Although research is an ongoing process, the existing body of evidence supports its potential to promote well-being.

2. Mechanisms of Action at the Cellular Level: A Symphony of Interactions

Jigsimur's power lies in its ability to interact with cells at the most fundamental level. Its diverse array of natural ingredients triggers a symphony of responses within the body, contributing to its multifaceted effects. For example, the anti-inflammatory properties of certain components can influence cellular pathways that regulate inflammation, while antioxidants neutralize harmful free radicals. These intricate

interactions create an environment that supports the body's natural processes.

3. Bridging Traditional Wisdom and Modern Science: A Unified Approach

The fusion of traditional wisdom and modern scientific understanding is a powerful alliance that enriches our perception of Jigsimur's effects. Science validates the insights of indigenous healers and offers a deeper understanding of how its ingredients impact the body. By uniting these two perspectives, we celebrate both the wisdom of ancient traditions and the advancements of contemporary research, acknowledging the harmony that emerges when nature and science collaborate.

The Dance of Knowledge: Weaving the Past with the Present

1. Validation Through Research: Scientific studies provide tangible evidence of Jigsimur's efficacy, offering insights into its potential benefits.

2. Unlocking Cellular Interactions: Understanding the cellular mechanisms through which Jigsimur exerts its effects unveils the intricate harmony of nature's compounds.

3. Ancient Meets Modern: The synergy between traditional wisdom and modern research enriches our comprehension of Jigsimur's role in improving well-being.

4. Ongoing Explorations: As science continues to evolve, further discoveries may illuminate even more facets of Jigsimur's impact on health and wellness.

5. A Comprehensive Perspective: The union of ancient knowledge and scientific inquiry enriches our understanding, allowing us to appreciate the complexity of Jigsimur's effects.

A Path of Illumination: Blending Wisdom and Knowledge

As we delve into the research and scientific insights surrounding Jigsimur, we embark on a journey of discovery that harmonizes traditional wisdom with modern understanding. The revelations of cellular interactions and the validation of its effectiveness through research guide us toward a deeper appreciation of Jigsimur's potential. With this newfound understanding, we step into the next phase of our exploration—exploring the real-life stories of transformation through Jigsimur's embrace.

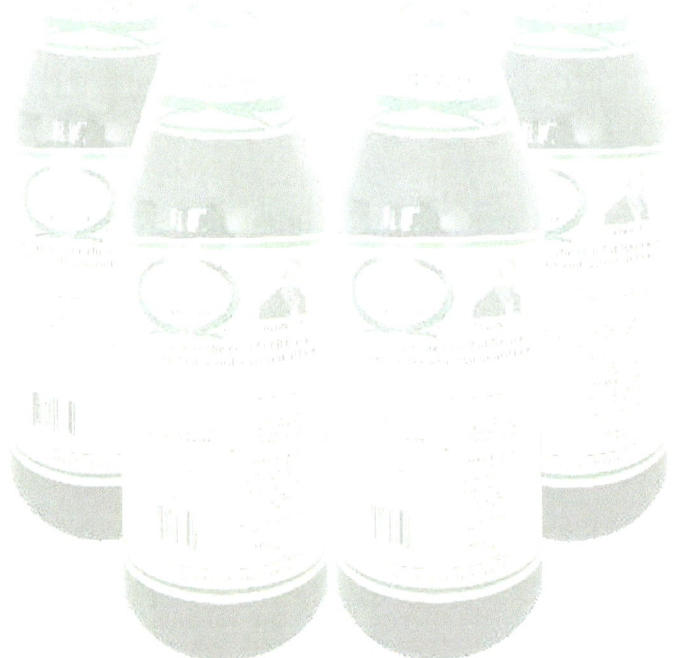

Chapter 8

Testimonials and Success Stories

Voices of Transformation: Real-Life Journeys with Jigsimur

In this chapter, the spotlight turns to the heartwarming tales of individuals whose lives have been touched by the power of Jigsimur. Through their firsthand experiences, we glimpse the diverse ways in which this natural treasure has inspired remarkable health transformations and improvements, transcending boundaries and resonating with the essence of holistic wellness.

1. Real-Life Experiences from Jigsimur Users: A Symphony of Voices

The stories within these pages are not mere narratives; they are the voices of individuals who have embarked on their wellness journeys with Jigsimur. They share their experiences, challenges, and triumphs—each a unique thread woven into the tapestry of transformation. These real-life accounts provide a glimpse into the spectrum of health issues that Jigsimur addresses, creating a testament to its versatile potential.

2. Varied Health Transformations and Improvements: A Kaleidoscope of Change

The narratives collected here tell of more than just health improvements; they speak of holistic transformations that encompass physical, emotional, and even spiritual well-being. Individuals share their journeys of finding relief from joint discomfort, experiencing enhanced digestive health, boosting immunity, and more. The power of Jigsimur shines through as lives are uplifted through a renewed sense of vitality and well-being.

Stories of Hope and Empowerment: Igniting the Flame of Change

1. From Challenges to Triumphs: The testimonials unveil the diverse health challenges that Jigsimur has addressed, showcasing the breadth of its potential.

2. A Tapestry of Transformations: Each story paints a vivid picture of personal growth, wellness enhancements, and newfound vitality.

3. A Ripple of Inspiration: These stories offer hope and inspire others to embark on their own journeys toward holistic wellness.

4. Elevating Quality of Life: The diverse improvements recounted in these testimonials touch upon multiple dimensions of well-being.

5. Empowerment through Experience: Jigsimur users' journeys underscore the empowerment that comes from embracing natural solutions for health.

An Odyssey of Well-Being: Testimonies That Illuminate the Path

The stories shared within these pages are a celebration of human resilience, the power of nature's remedies, and the boundless potential of the body's innate healing abilities. They serve as beacons of inspiration for those seeking a path to holistic well-being. As we proceed to the concluding chapters of this ebook, let the transformative experiences of Jigsimur users guide us toward a deeper appreciation of its profound impact.

Chapter 9

Exploring Alternative Medicine

Beyond the Conventional: Jigsimur's Role in Holistic Health and Healing

In this chapter, we venture into the realm of alternative medicine—a path that aligns with the principles of holistic health and embraces the wisdom of traditional remedies. By examining Jigsimur in the context of this broader approach, we uncover its potential to complement conventional treatments and offer a holistic perspective on well-being.

1. Jigsimur in the Context of Holistic Health: Nurturing Mind, Body, and Spirit

Alternative medicine is grounded in the philosophy of treating the whole person—mind, body, and spirit. Jigsimur's natural composition resonates with this philosophy, addressing not only physical symptoms but also contributing to emotional and spiritual well-being. By offering a multifaceted approach, Jigsimur aligns seamlessly with the principles of holistic health, fostering harmony across various dimensions of existence.

2. Comparing Traditional Remedies with Conventional Treatments: A Balanced Perspective

The world of health and wellness is rich with options, each with its own merits. Traditional remedies and conventional treatments are two distinct paths, and their benefits can often be complementary.

While conventional medicine excels in acute care and advanced interventions, traditional remedies like Jigsimur excel in improving preventive measures, supporting chronic condition management, and fostering overall well-being. It's important to approach this comparison with an open mind, recognizing that both avenues supply to the mosaic of health care.

Harmony and Balance: Merging Ancient Wisdom with Modern Understanding

1. Holistic Synergy: Jigsimur's holistic approach resonates with the principles of alternative medicine, embracing the interconnectedness of mind, body, and spirit.

2. A Tapestry of Options: Traditional remedies and conventional treatments each have their place, contributing to a comprehensive approach to well-being.

3. Informed Choices: The path to health is unique for each individual. By considering a range of options, you empower yourself to make informed decisions.

4. Bridging Wisdom and Advancements: Combining traditional wisdom with modern understanding creates a balanced and harmonious approach to health.

5. Embracing Diversity: By embracing alternative medicine and traditional remedies, you open doors to a diverse array of possibilities for well-being.

A Holistic Spectrum: Blending Pathways to Wellness

As we explore the realm of alternative medicine and its alignment with holistic health, we step into a world where ancient wisdom and contemporary understanding converge. By considering the role of Jigsimur within this broader context, we illuminate the diverse tapestry of options available for cultivating well-being. The following chapters continue our journey, delving into the intricate connection between Jigsimur, the human body, and the pursuit of lasting health and vitality.

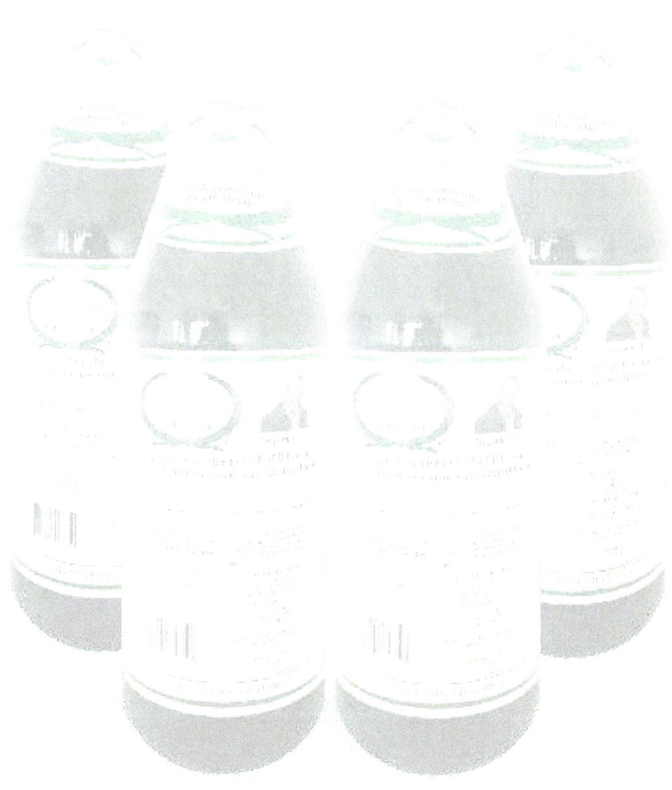

Chapter 10

Navigating the Market

Choosing Wisely: A Guide to Navigating the World of Jigsimur Products

In this chapter, we delve into the practical realm of navigating the market to ensure that you are making informed decisions when selecting Jigsimur products. As the demand for natural remedies grows, it's essential to equip yourself with the knowledge needed to identify genuine, quality products that align with your health and wellness goals.

1. Identifying Genuine Jigsimur Products: Trustworthy Sources

The authenticity of Jigsimur products is paramount for experiencing its true benefits. To ensure you're purchasing genuine Jigsimur, seek out reputable sources. Look for authorized distributors or official websites affiliated with Jigsimur. These sources are more likely to offer products that adhere to the highest standards of quality and authenticity.

2. Recognizing Quality and Authenticity: Certifications and Labels

Genuine Jigsimur products often carry certifications and labels that validate their quality and authenticity. Look for markers such as quality assurance seals, organic certifications, and manufacturing standards that reflect a commitment to producing products of high integrity. These certifications offer peace of mind that you're investing in a product that meets stringent criteria.

3. Selecting the Right Form: Liquid, Capsules, or Powder

Jigsimur is available in various forms, each offering distinct advantages. The choice between liquid, capsules, or powder depends on your personal preferences and lifestyle. Liquid forms often allow for more rapid absorption, capsules offer convenience for on-the-go use, and powders can

be versatile for mixing into beverages or foods. Consider your preferences and how each form aligns with your daily routine

A Journey of Informed Choices: Navigating the Market with Confidence

1. Research and Verify: Ensure you're purchasing Jigsimur from reputable sources, such as authorized distributors or official websites.

2. Seek Certifications: Look for certifications and quality assurance labels that validate the product's authenticity and quality.

3. Consider Form Preferences: Choose between liquid, capsules, or powder based on your lifestyle and how you prefer to incorporate Jigsimur into your routine.

4. Read Reviews: Feedback from other users can provide insights into the quality and effectiveness of different products.

5. Consult Professionals: If unsure, consult healthcare professionals or experts in natural medicine for guidance.

An Empowered Approach: Making Informed Choices

As you navigate the market for Jigsimur products, you're taking a proactive step towards your well-being. By seeking authenticity, quality, and the right form that suits your lifestyle, you're ensuring that your journey with Jigsimur is rooted in trust and effectiveness. With the tools provided in this chapter, you're poised to make informed choices that align with your health and wellness aspirations. The following chapters continue our exploration, delving into the practical aspects of incorporating Jigsimur into your daily life.

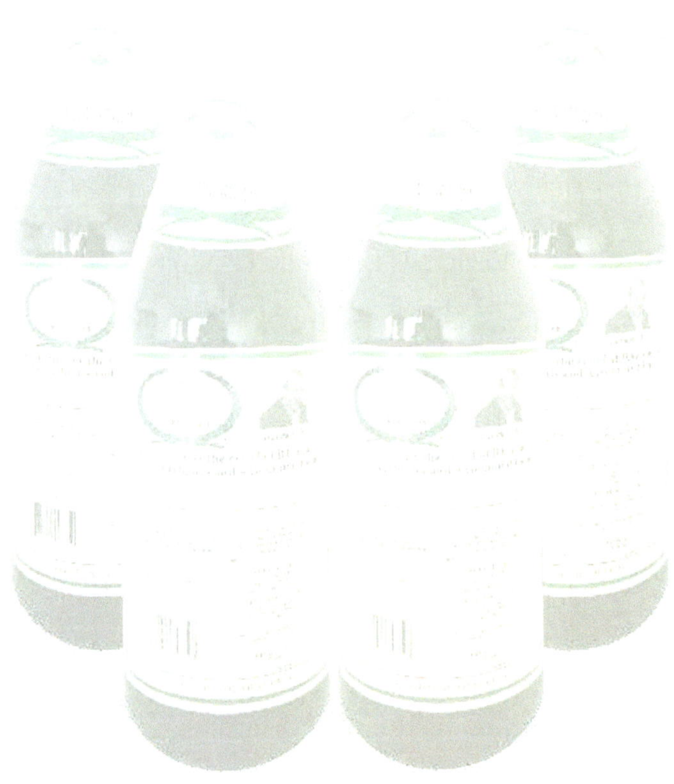

Chapter 11

Future of Jigsimur

Charting a Path of Promise: The Evolution of Jigsimur in Health and Wellness

In this chapter, we cast our gaze toward the future, envisioning the exciting possibilities that lie ahead for Jigsimur. As this natural treasure continues to inspire health and well-being, we explore its potential for deeper scientific validation, global recognition, accessibility, and the crucial ethical considerations that will shape its sustainable journey.

1. Potential for Further Scientific Validation: Unveiling New Dimensions

The journey of Jigsimur is an ongoing exploration, and the horizon holds promise for further scientific validation. As research methodologies advance, the potential exists to uncover even more facets of Jigsimur's effects on health and wellness. Future studies might reveal intricate mechanisms of action, delve into its potential in addressing emerging health challenges, and strengthen its position as a valuable component of holistic health practices.

2. Global Recognition and Accessibility: A Worldwide Wellness Movement

The essence of Jigsimur's benefits knows no boundaries. As awareness spreads, so too does its accessibility to people worldwide. With growing recognition within the global health and wellness community, Jigsimur could become a sought-after natural solution that transcends cultures and backgrounds. This journey toward global recognition paves the way for greater availability, enabling more individuals to experience its transformative potential.

3. Ethical Considerations and Sustainability: Nurturing Nature's Gift Responsibly

As Jigsimur gains traction, it's crucial to remain rooted in ethical considerations and sustainability. Responsible sourcing, fair trade practices, and the preservation of the source ingredients are paramount. Upholding the well-being of the communities involved in its creation aligns with the principles of holistic health and ensures the perpetuity of this precious natural treasure.

A Vision of Possibility: Shaping the Destiny of Jigsimur

1. Advancing Knowledge: The future holds the promise of deeper insights into Jigsimur's effects through cutting-edge scientific research.

2. Spreading Wellness: Jigsimur's journey toward global recognition paves the way for its accessibility to a wider audience seeking natural solutions.

3. A Legacy of Responsibility: Ethical considerations and sustainability practices safeguard the integrity of Jigsimur and the communities involved.

4. Navigating the Future: As Jigsimur evolves, its path will be guided by principles of authenticity, integrity, and holistic well-being.

5. Embracing the Unseen: The future unfolds with the potential to reveal new dimensions of Jigsimur's impact and its role in the well-being landscape.

A Tapestry of Promise: Envisioning Jigsimur's Continued Impact

As we conclude this chapter, we stand at the crossroads of anticipation. The future of Jigsimur is rich with possibility—further scientific validation, global recognition, and a commitment to ethical practices that resonate with its natural essence. By looking forward, we celebrate the ongoing journey of Jigsimur and the integral role it will play in the wellness journeys of countless individuals around the world. The concluding chapters of this ebook bring us closer to fully embracing the transformative potential of Jigsimur in our lives.

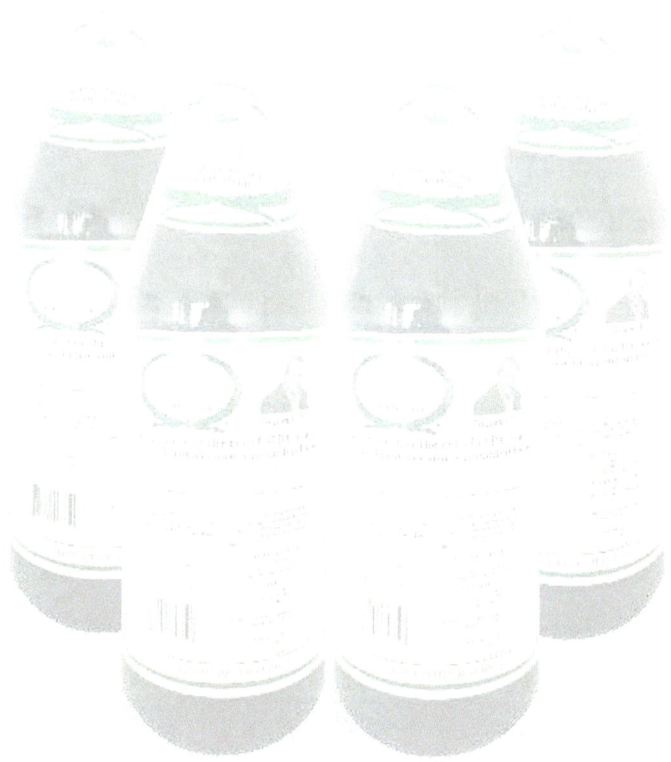

Conclusion

Embracing the Journey of Jigsimur

A Tapestry Woven in Nature: Reflecting on the Path of Discovery

As we reach the conclusion of this journey through the world of "Jigsimur: Nature's Treasure for Health and Wellness," we find ourselves immersed in the rich tapestry of wisdom, science, and transformation that Jigsimur has to offer. Throughout these pages, we've embarked on a voyage that bridges ancient traditions with modern understanding, revealing the profound impact of a natural treasure on the canvas of holistic well-being.

A Holistic Odyssey: Celebrating Nature's Bounty

Our exploration of Jigsimur's origins, ingredients, mechanisms of action, and the real-life stories of those who have embraced its potential has unveiled the remarkable depth and breadth of its influence. From digestive health to joint vitality, from immune support to emotional well-being, Jigsimur's effects resonate through multiple dimensions of existence, reminding us that well-being is a holistic endeavor.

Nature and Science in Harmony: A Symphony of Possibility

The harmonious dance of traditional wisdom and modern scientific validation echoes the intricate interplay between nature and human understanding. As we journeyed through research, testimonials, and the potential for the future, we witnessed how Jigsimur seamlessly blends ancient insights with contemporary insights, creating a symphony of possibility for enhanced health and vitality.

An Empowering Choice: Navigating Wellness with Wisdom

The decision to embrace Jigsimur as part of your wellness journey is a testament to your commitment to holistic health. By incorporating its

potential into your daily routine, you're embracing the wisdom of nature and the advancements of science, aligning your path with the principles of balance, well-being, and empowerment.

Beyond the Pages: Embracing the Future

As we close this chapter of exploration, remember that the journey of Jigsimur extends far beyond these pages. It continues with every choice you make to nurture your well-being, to seek authentic products, and to integrate its potential into your life. The future holds the promise of deeper insights, wider accessibility, and an enduring commitment to ethical practices that safeguard its source.

A Journey of Transformation: Your Tale Unfolds

The narrative of Jigsimur is not confined to these words; it extends into the stories of those who have experienced its transformative touch. With each success story, with each pursuit of well-being, the tale of Jigsimur grows richer and more vibrant, a testament to the profound union between nature and the human spirit.

Onward and Upward: The Quest Continues

As you move forward, may the wisdom of Jigsimur guide your path, may its potential inspire your journey, and may the harmony between tradition and modernity illuminate your pursuit of holistic health and wellness. As the chapters of your life unfold, let the legacy of Jigsimur be a source of empowerment, a beacon of authenticity, and a reminder that nature's treasures hold boundless potential for well-being.

Thank you for joining us on this voyage through "Jigsimur: Nature's Treasure for Health and Wellness." May your path be illuminated by the knowledge and inspiration you've gained, and may your well-being journey be as transformative and vibrant as the legacy of Jigsimur itself.

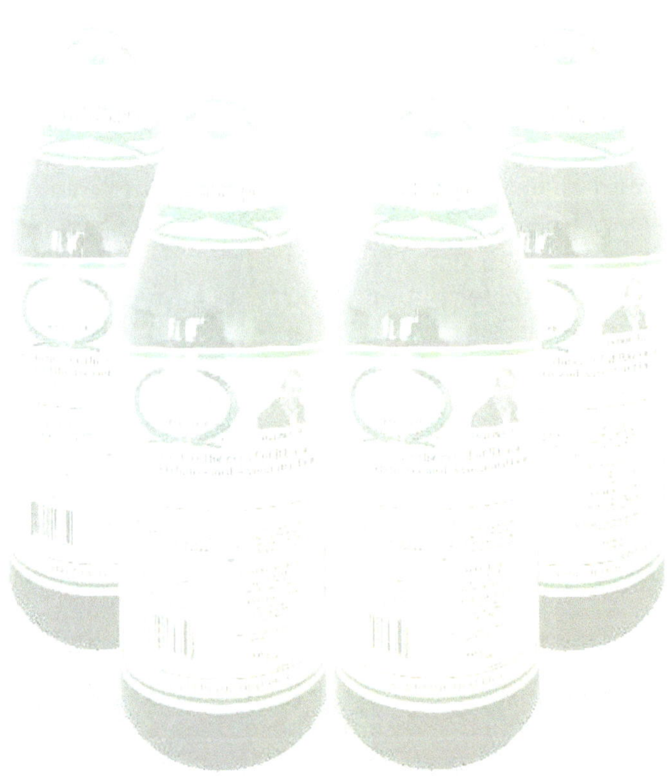

For Marketing Purposes Only

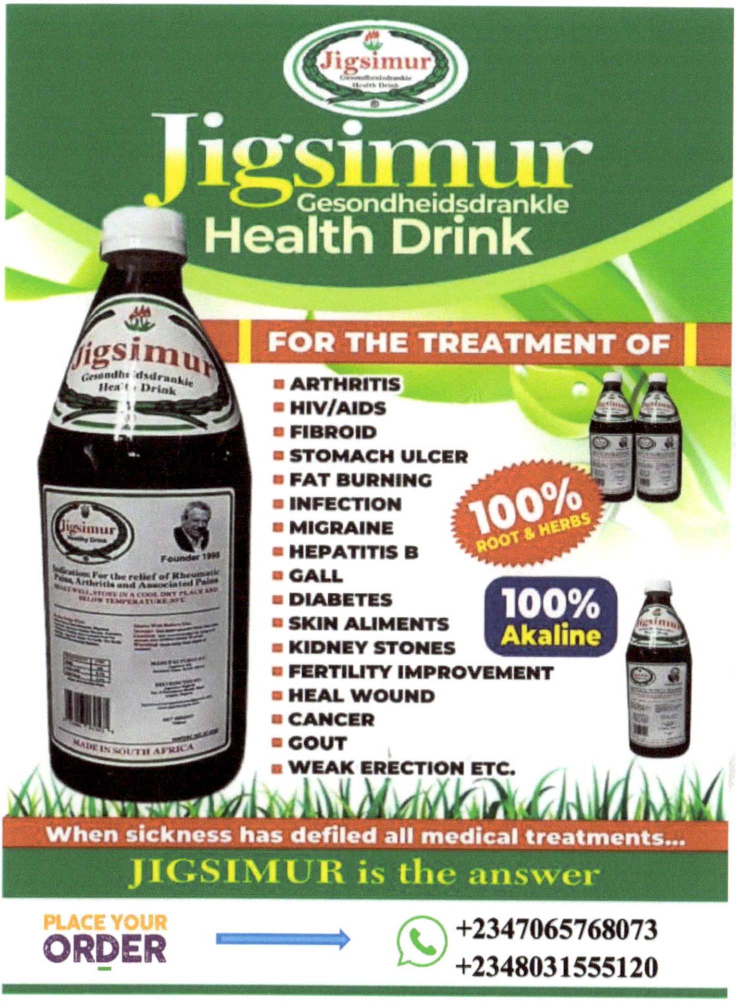

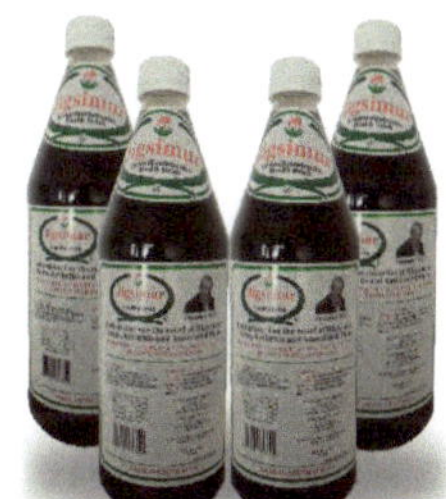